Can I eat a banana peel?

World Book
answers YOUR questions
- about -
food and eating

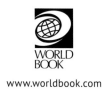

WORLD
BOOK

www.worldbook.com

Why do cakes get fluffy when they're baked?

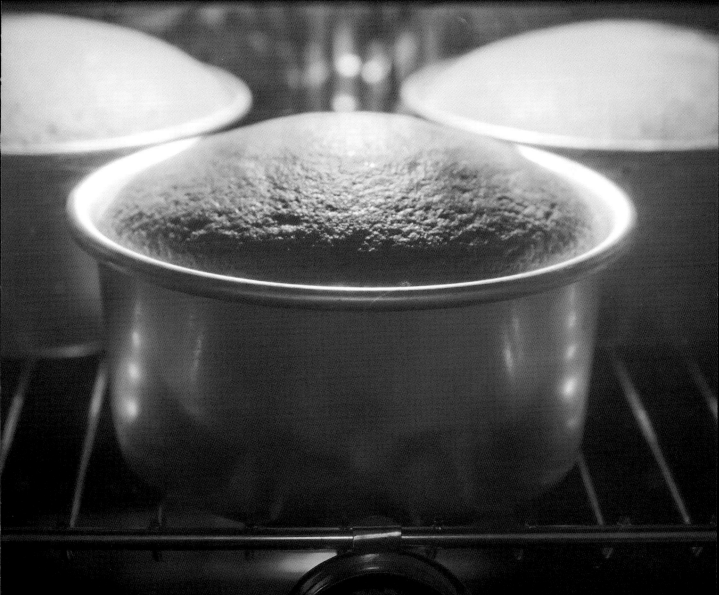

The secret ingredient:
air.

Good bakers do the little things: making sure the butter and eggs are at room temperature, whisking them gently with the sugar, and adding the flour through a sifter. All that work, along with a little baking powder or baking soda, adds millions of tiny air bubbles to the batter. Gas expands when it's heated, so the cake rises and takes on a fluffy texture.

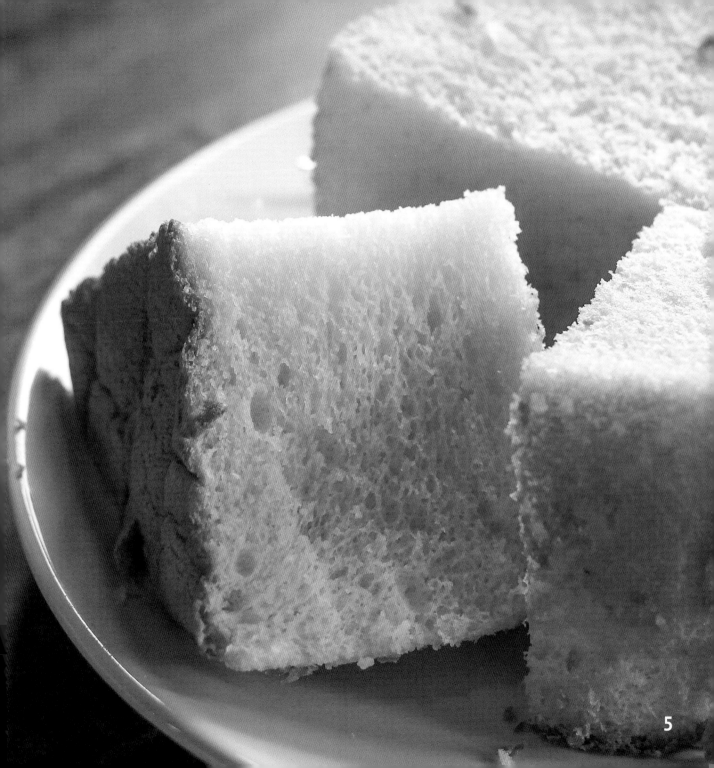

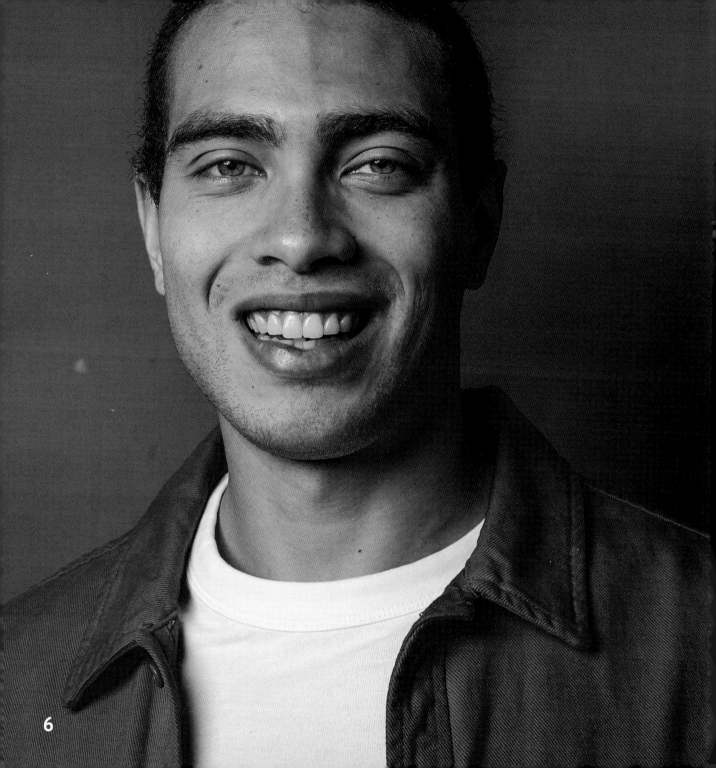

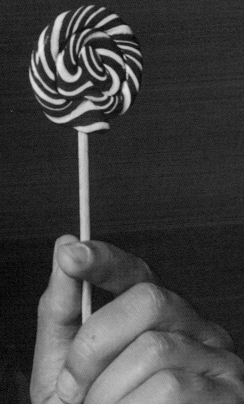

Who invented candy?

The same people who invented the
365-day calendar, hieroglyphics, and papyrus:

the ancient Egyptians.

These are all wonderful achievements,
and chief among them is candy. Three
thousand years ago, ancient Egyptians made
confections by mixing fruits and nuts with
honey. People in ancient India became the
first to make candy with sugar cane.
Thanks to these ancient peoples for
making all of our lives a bit less sour.
Well, unless we're eating sour candies.

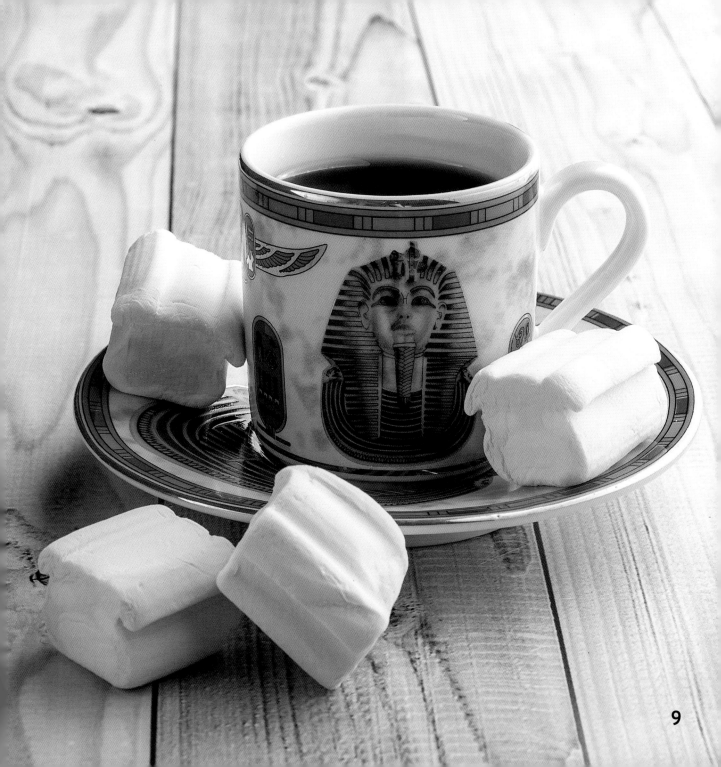

Why does cilantro taste like soap?

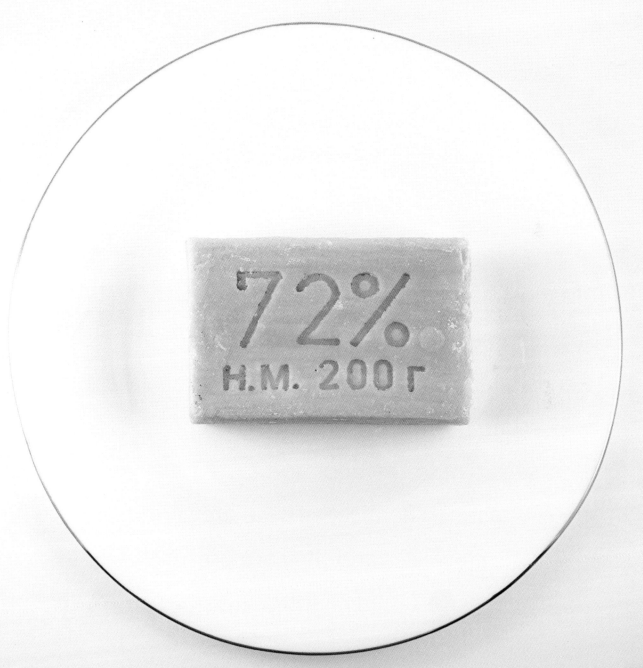

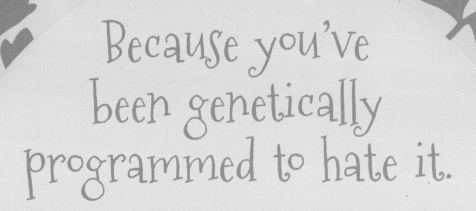

Because you've been genetically programmed to hate it.

To most people, cilantro has a light, citrusy flavor. But to some people, it tastes soapy and rotten. Yuck. Genes might be to blame for this flavor difference. Certain groups of genes make people really sensitive to the odor and taste of soapy-tasting chemicals. These are called *aldehydes* and they are present in cilantro.

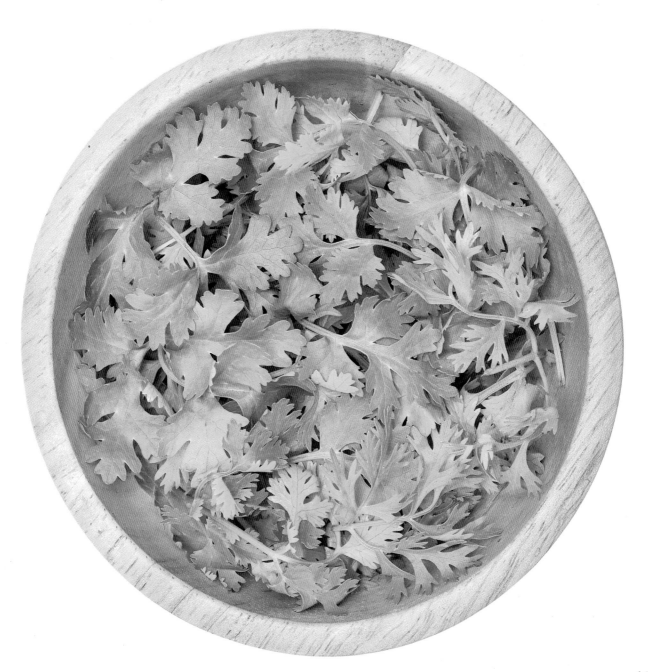

Can I eat a banana peel?

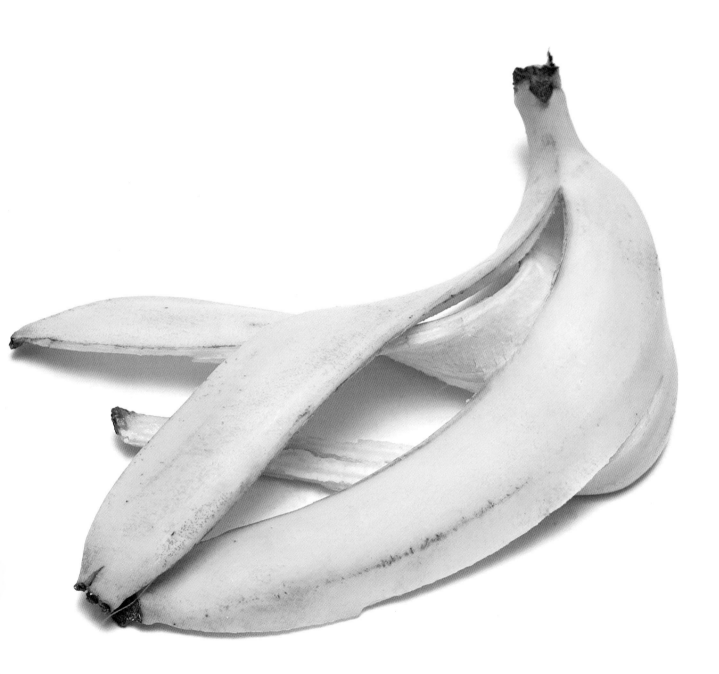

15

The bitter taste and tough texture

might not be **apeeling,** but you *can* eat a banana peel. It has such vitamins and minerals as potassium and amino acids. Plus, it's high in fiber. And, one other thing: when you eat your peel, you save someone from a very embarrassing slip.

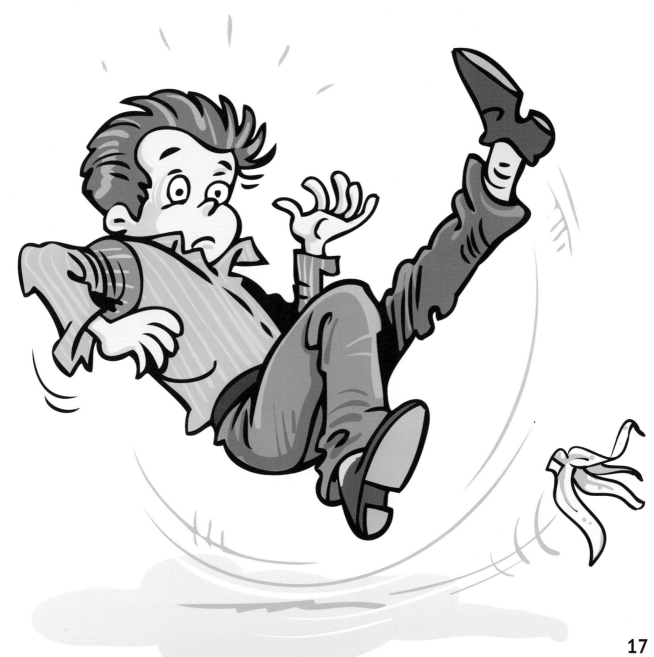

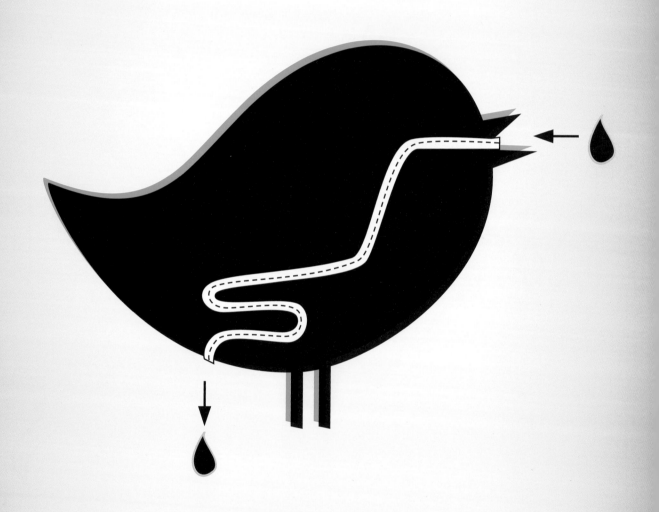

Why do birds digest?

The same reason we digest: to fuel our bodies.

Birds are warm-blooded. That means they keep their bodies at a constant, high temperature. Birds need food to do this. Lots of food. They spend most of their waking hours looking for food to digest.

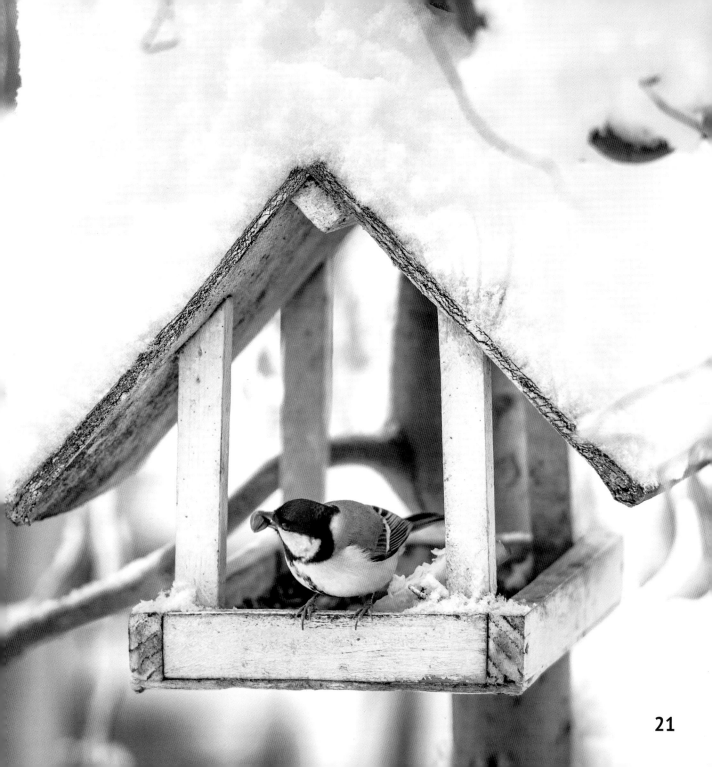

Why is gum chewy?

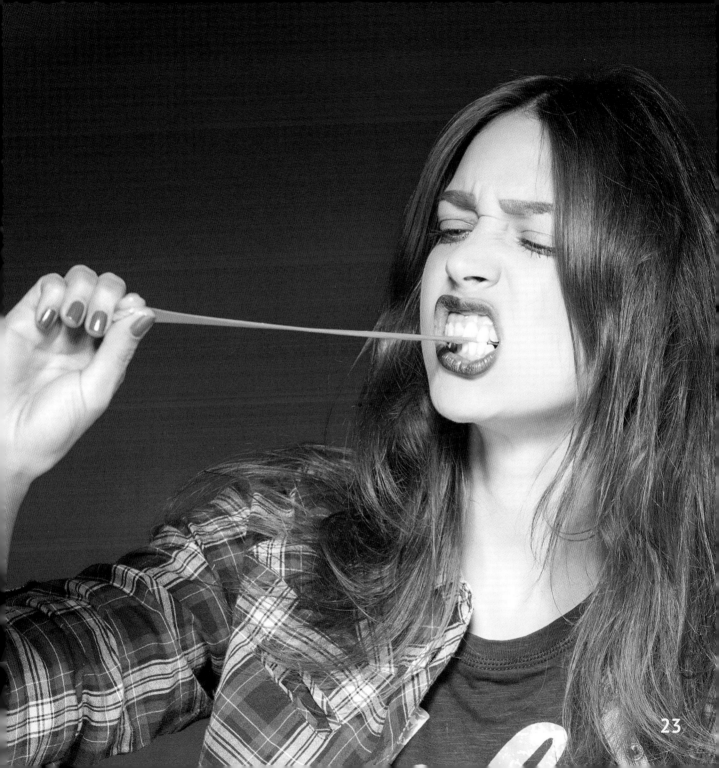

Gum is chewy because of gum.

We're not being *facetious*—a fancy word for being funny when you're not supposed to. Gum base is an ingredient that makes gum chewy and holds the flavorings and other ingredients. Gum base is made up of waxes and sticky stuff from plants and trees.

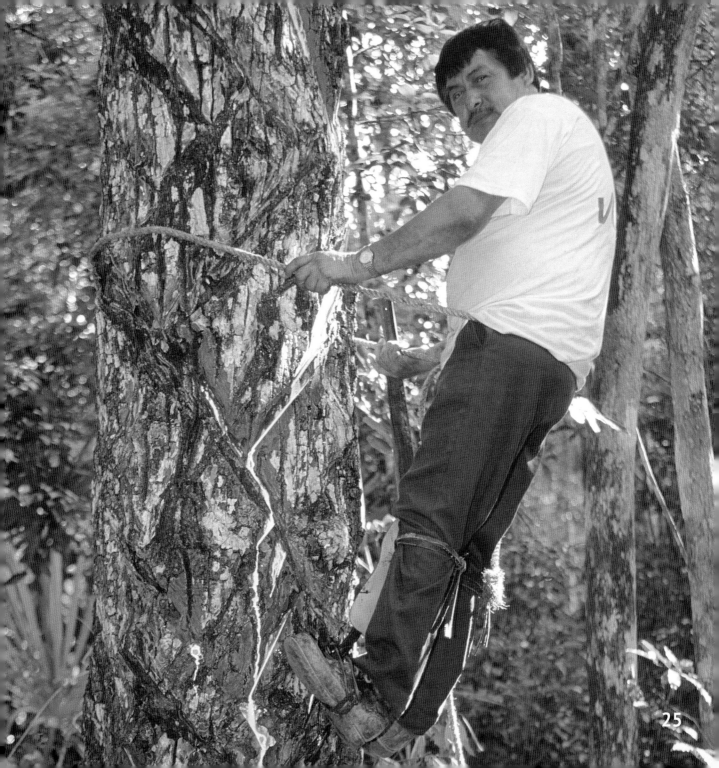

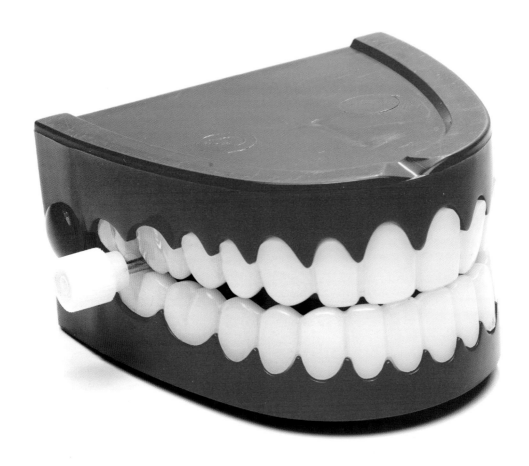

What are teeth made of?

Special tissues called pulp, dentin, cementum, and enamel.

Have you ever heard the phrase, "It's what's on the inside that counts"? Well, **tooth be told,** this doesn't really apply to teeth. The outer coating of enamel is where the rubber meets the road—or where the tooth meets the food. Enamel is the hardest tissue in the body, but we throw a lot at it: apples, popcorn, braces, sports equipment, and candy—lots of candy. Be sure to take care of your teeth by cleaning them, getting dental checkups, and eating nutritious foods.

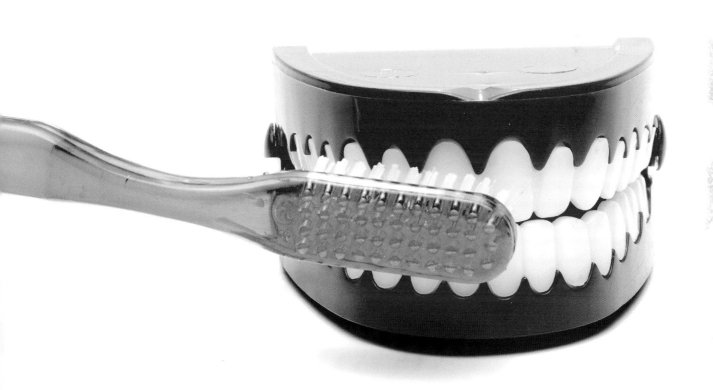

Where did the apricot get its name?

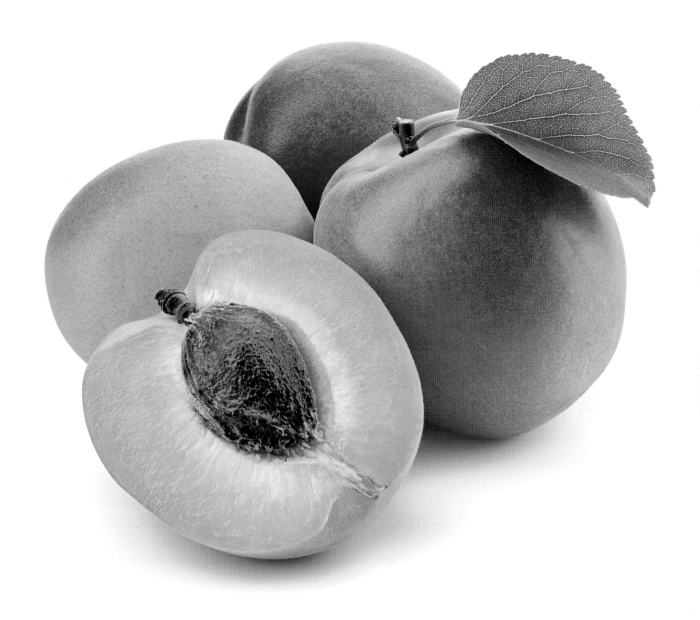

In the produce section of a market in either Iran or Turkey.

Those countries are the chief world producers of apricots. In truth, *apricot* ultimately comes from Latin words meaning *early-ripening fruit.*

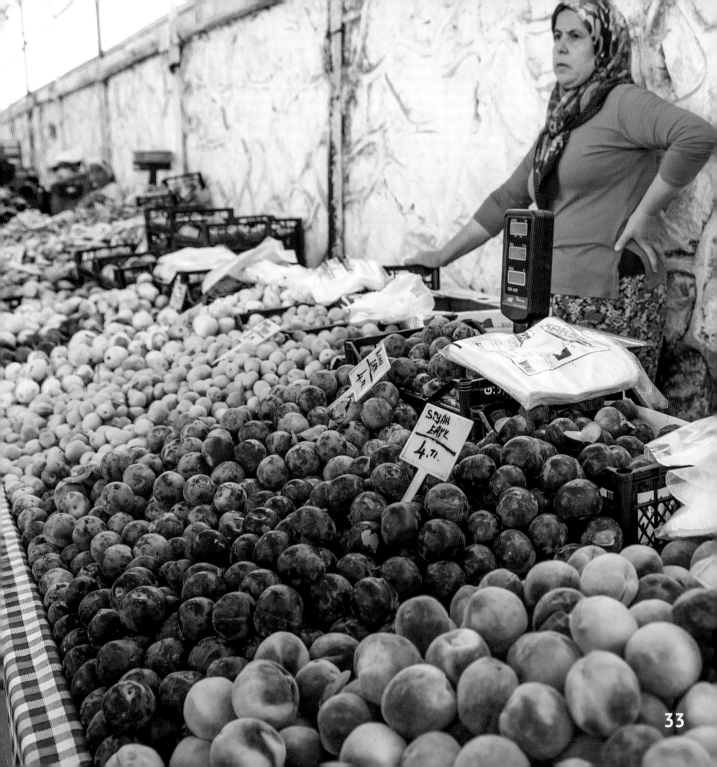

Does space food taste good?

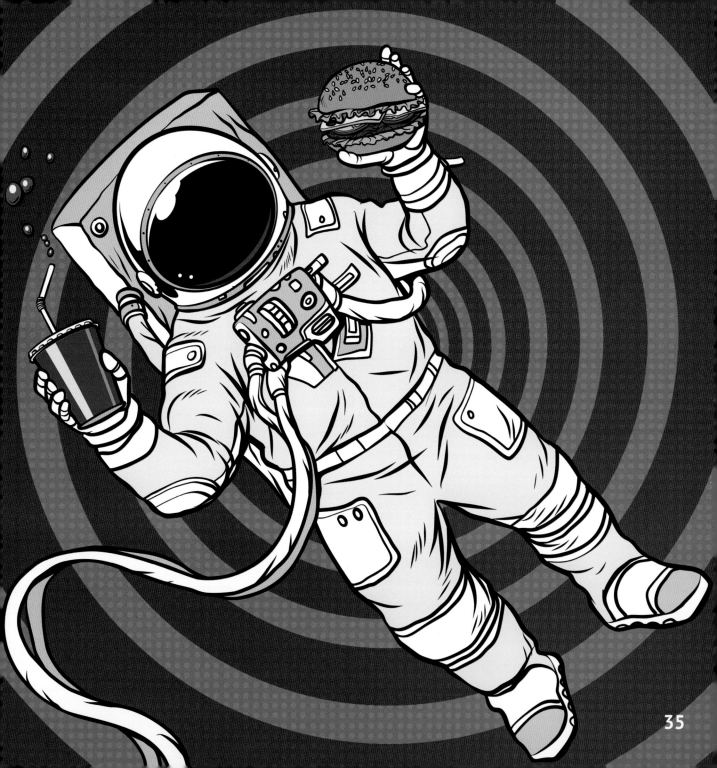

For an
astronaut to have
the right food in space,

she has to **planet.** Some foods have to be dried,

and others have to be liquefied. Salt and pepper,

for instance, can't be in their regular

form of teeny-tiny sprinkles because they might

float away. Does space food taste as good

as a home-cooked meal? I've never

heard an astronaut say so!

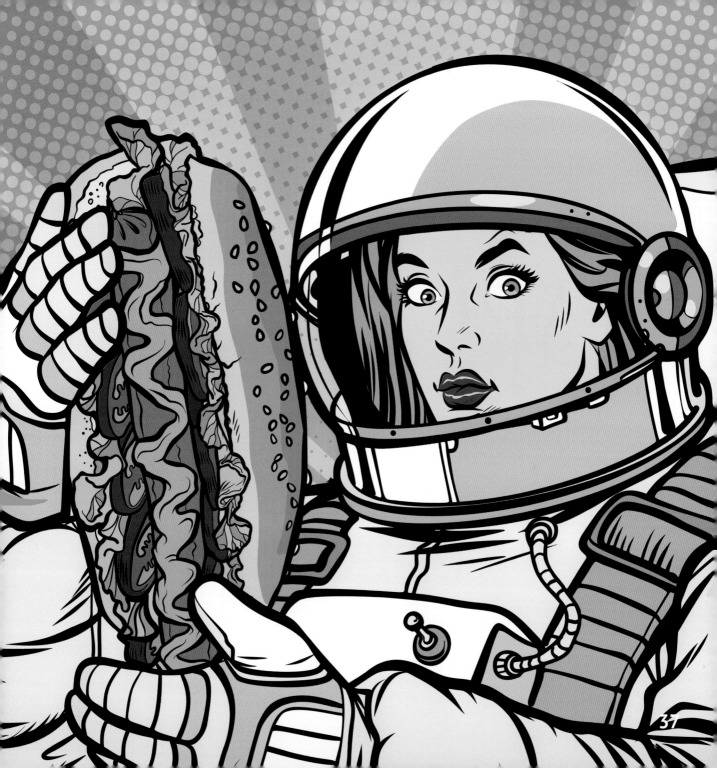

Do humans really swallow 8 spiders a year while they are sleeping?

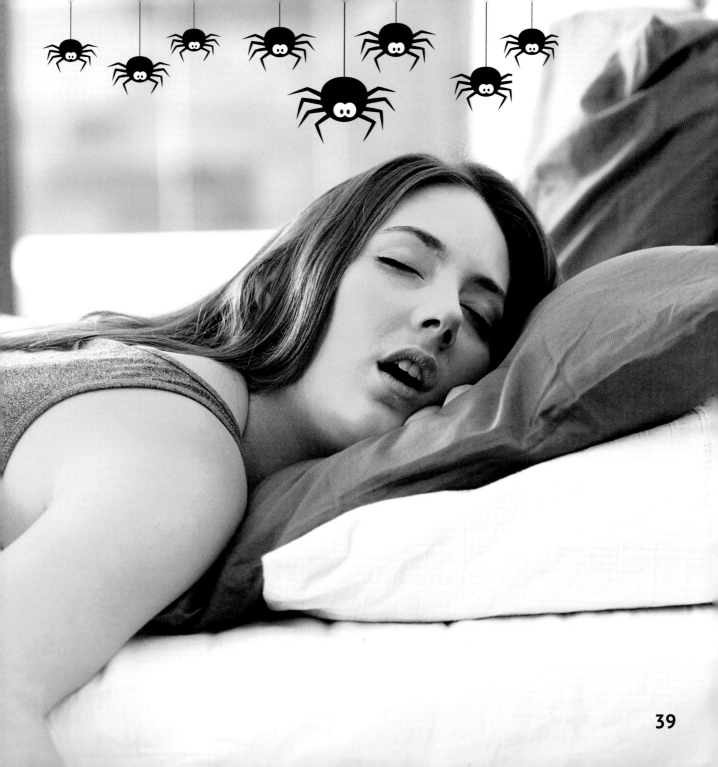

39

Nah.

Did you read that on the **web?** Sleeping people do not swallow eight spiders a year. Spiders use vibrations to sense danger. And when humans sleep, they are basically one big vibration. Humans breathe, snore, and toss and turn in their sleep. All those vibrations would scare spiders away. Also, a spider might get stuck in all your drool.

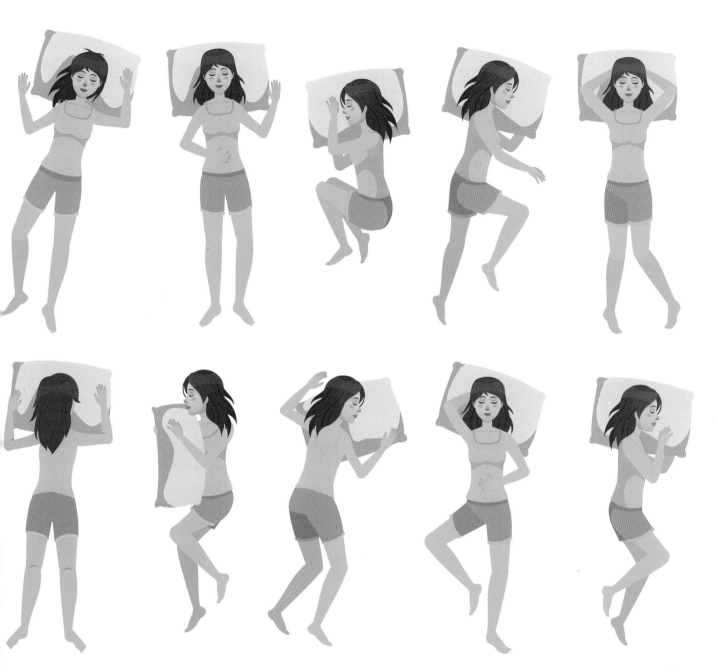

41

What is caffeine?

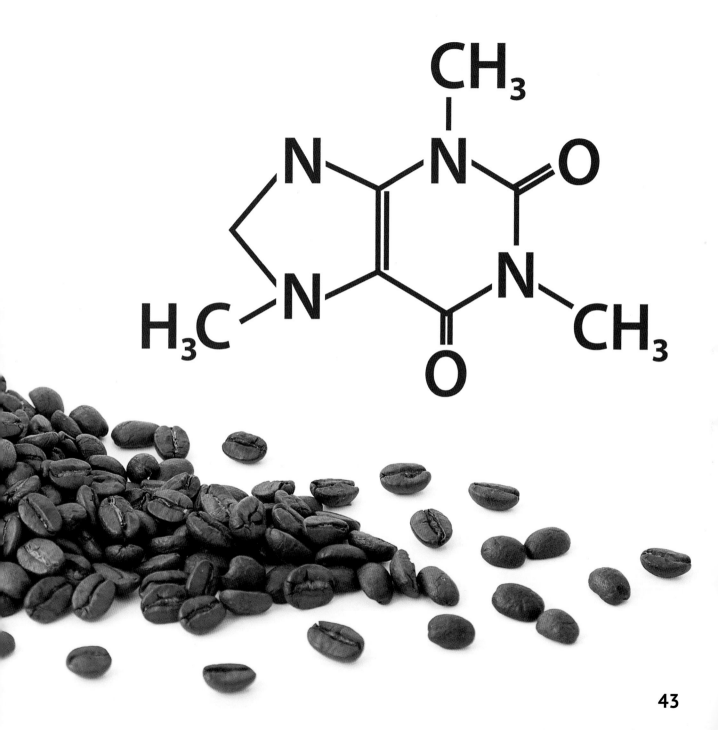

Caffeine is a slightly bitter solid that doesn't smell like anything.

You might be thinking, "What? Caffeine smells like hazelnut coffee or Earl Grey tea." Although caffeine is

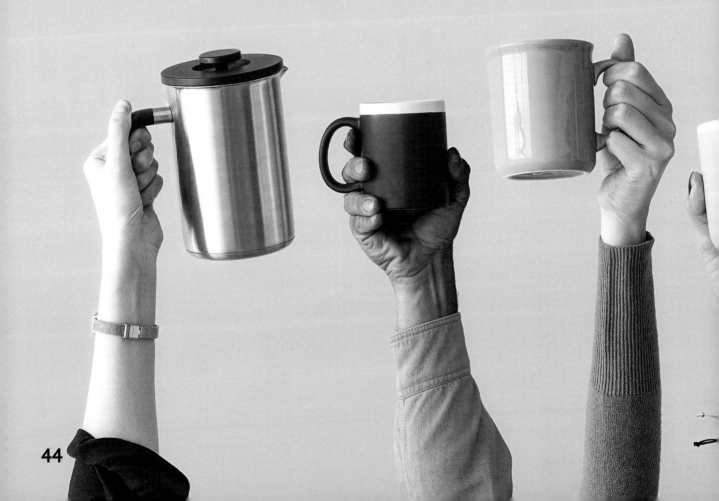

in those things, the caffeine itself doesn't smell like anything. Caffeine is a stimulant, which means that it gives you a **latte** energy. But when you have too much caffeine, you become nervous and jittery.

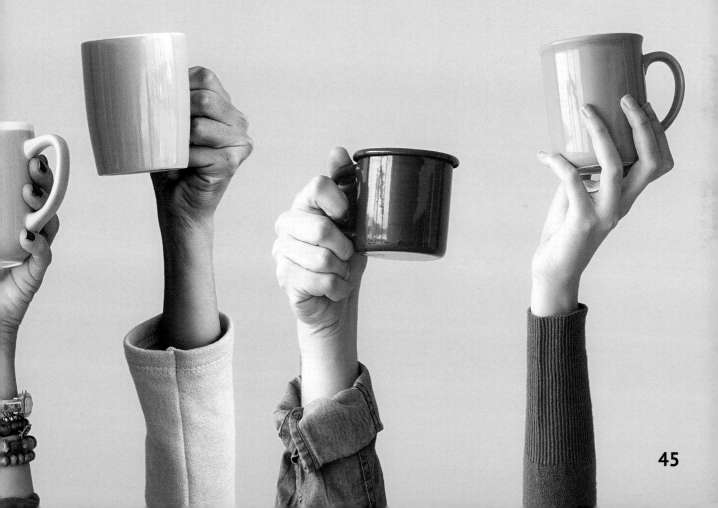

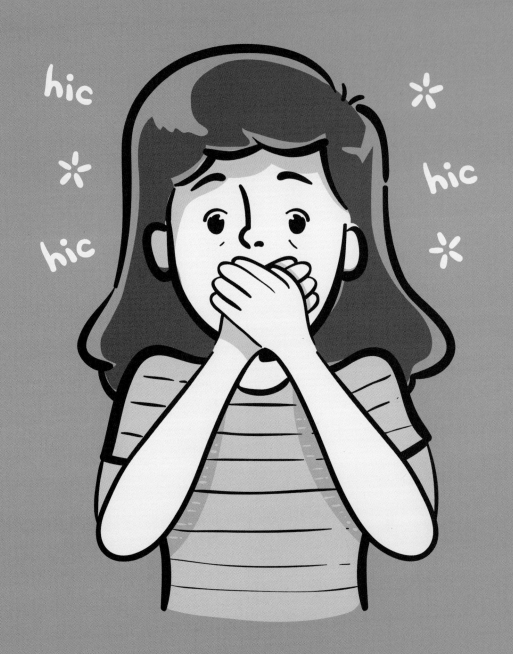

46

Why do we hiccup?

Because of a spasm in the diaphragm.

That difficult-to-spell word is a powerful muscle that lies at the base of the chest cavity. When the diaphragm suddenly contracts, the muscles in the chest and abdomen shake. Then, a part of your throat called the epiglottis closes. This creates the "hic" sound. A man named Charles Osborne had hiccups for more than 60 years. He hiccupped an estimated 430 million times in his lifetime.

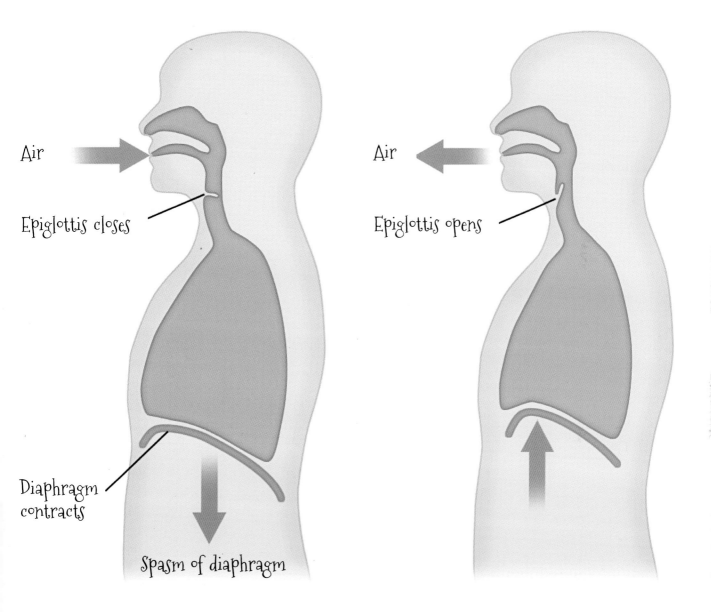

Air

Epiglottis closes

Diaphragm contracts

Spasm of diaphragm

Air

Epiglottis opens

What's a tongue twister?

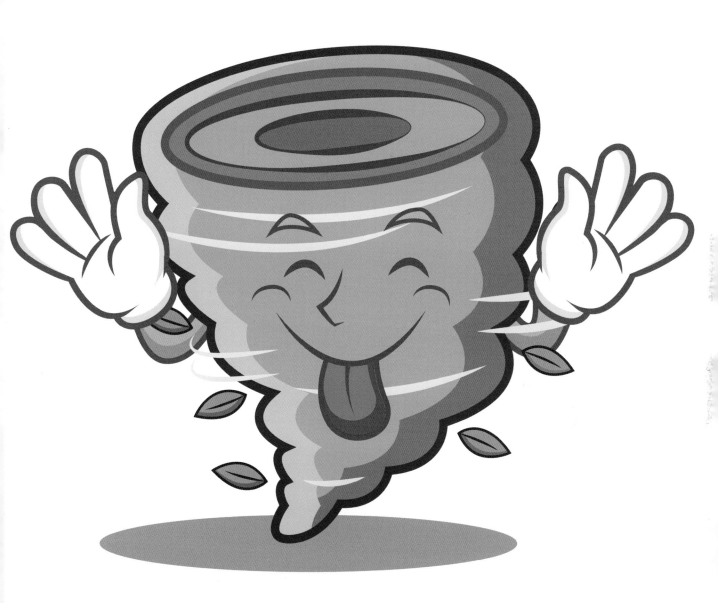

A tongue twister is a verse that's hard to say, like:

"Peter Piper picked a peck of pickled peppers."

What the **peck** did he need them for, anyway?

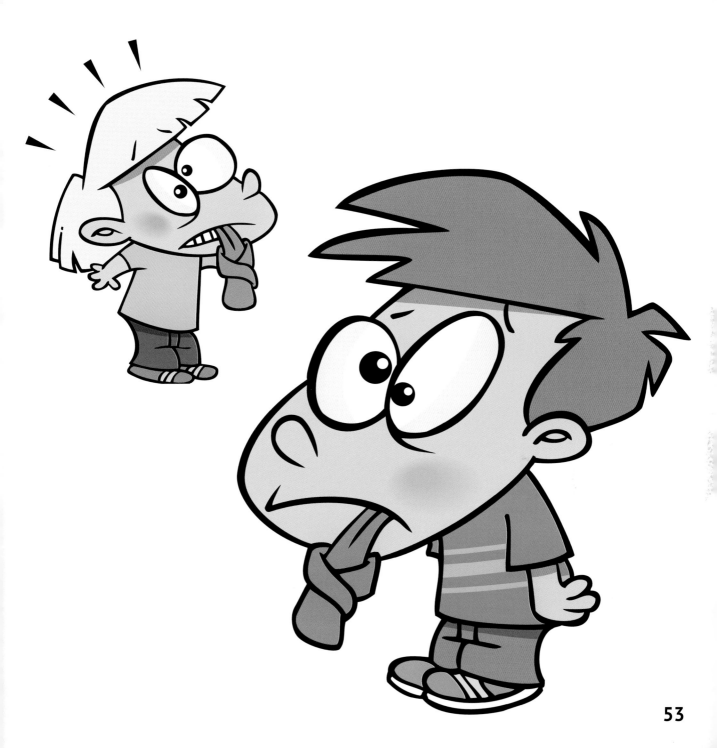

53

How good is lava at popping popcorn?

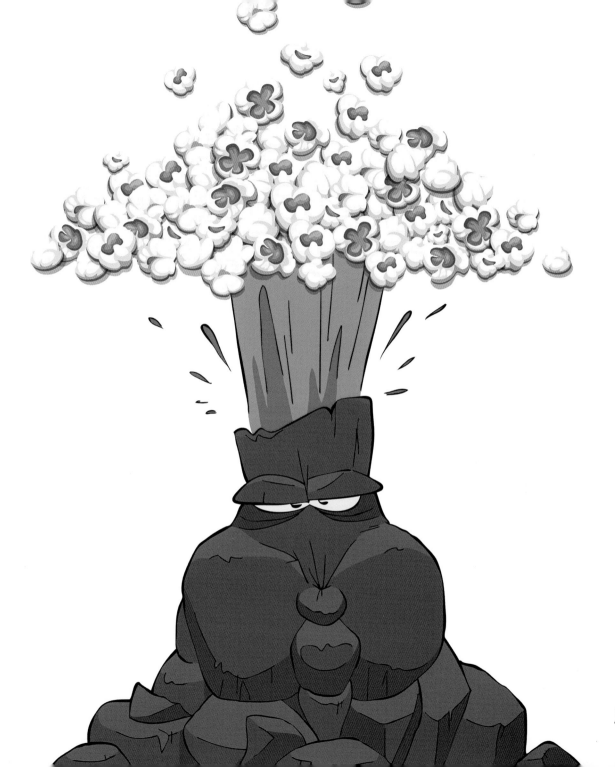

Do you love that burnt popcorn smell?

If you do, you should pop your popcorn with lava. The ideal temperature to pop popcorn is 360 °F (180 °C). Lava can be 2,200 °F (1,200 °C) when it erupts onto the surface. And you thought spicy-cheese or buffalo flavoring was hot.

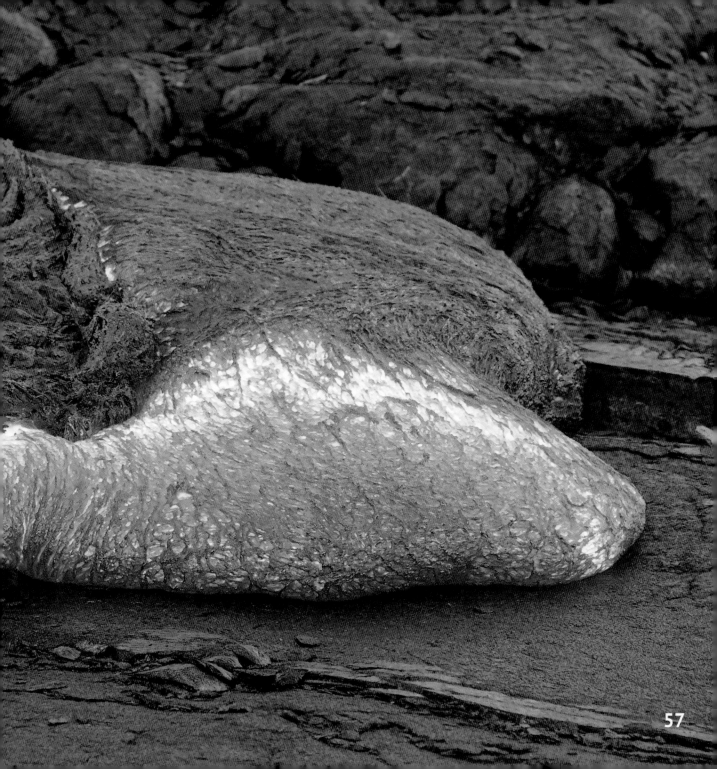

Why do lemons taste sour?

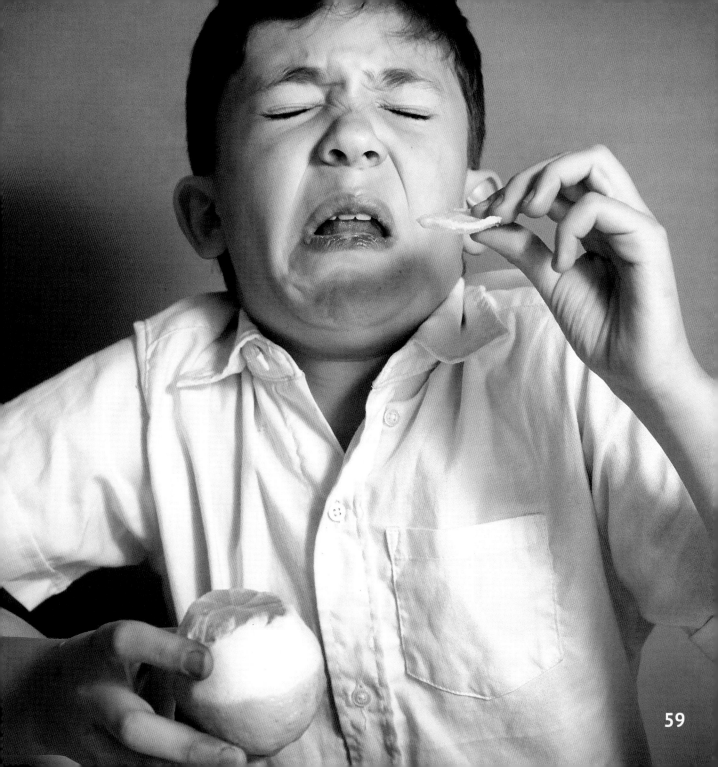

Because they think it's funny

when we pucker up our faces.

The sour stuff is actually citric acid.

The more citric acid, the funnier

the lemon thinks we look.

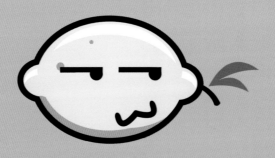

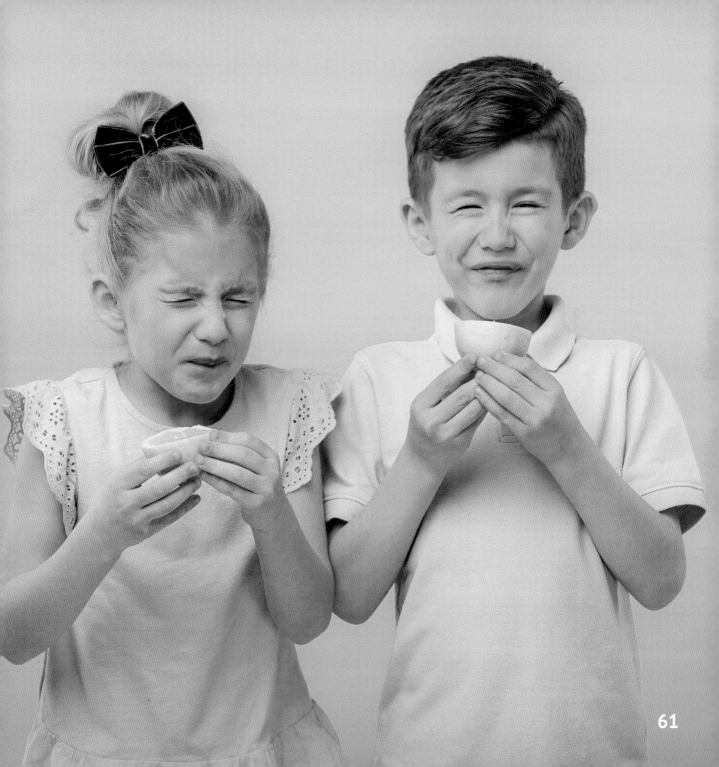

What is a food chain?

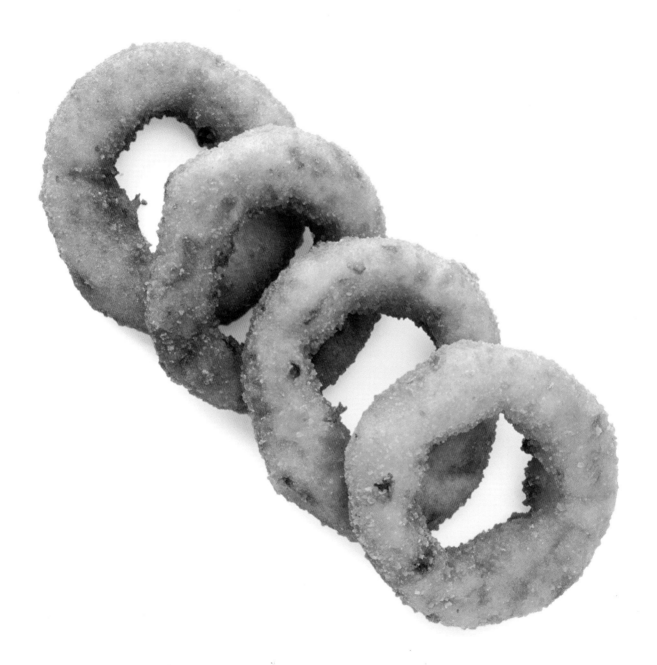

If you're thinking a food chain is a chain of interlocking onion rings,

we like where your head is at. But that's not
a food chain—it's a culinary masterpiece.
A food chain is a model of how energy in the
form of food passes from one organism to another.
A simple food chain might include a worm,
a fish, and a bigger fish.

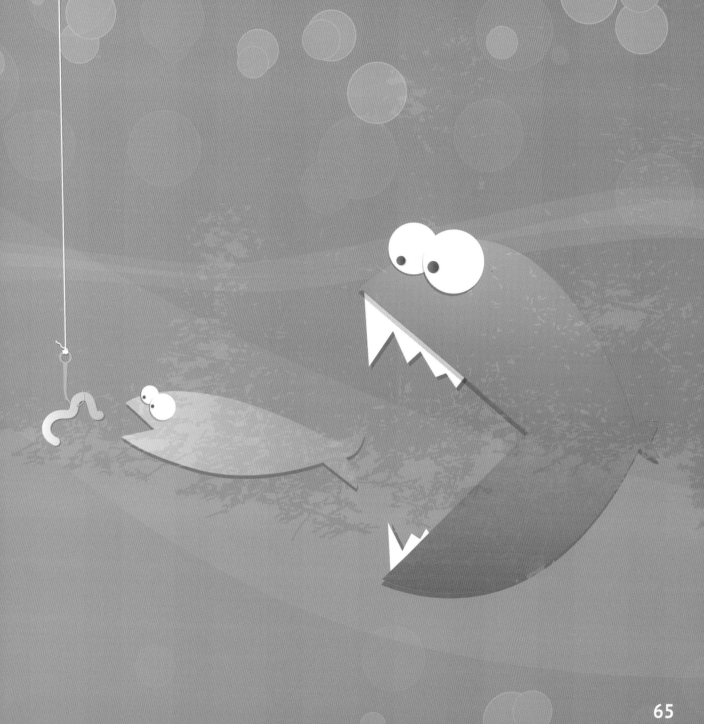

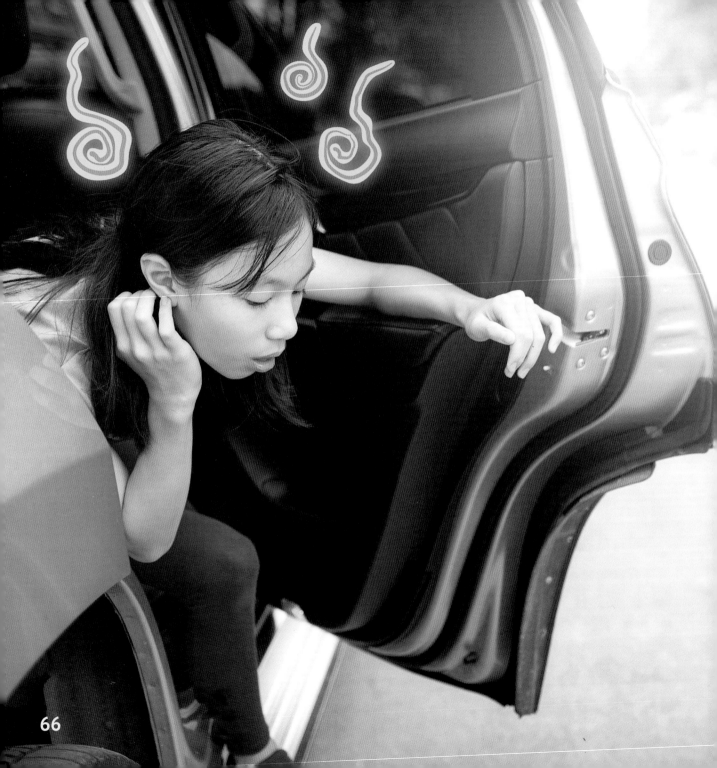

Why do we vomit our food out?

For all sorts of reasons.

We might get sick from food poisoning.
We might feel sick from the stomach flu.
We might have accidentally grabbed a
handful of chocolate-covered espresso
beans thinking they were raisins and, upon
crunching them, thought they tasted so
horrible that we immediately threw up on
an adult in a really fancy restaurant... or
something like that. Our bodies throw up
food that they want nothing to do with.

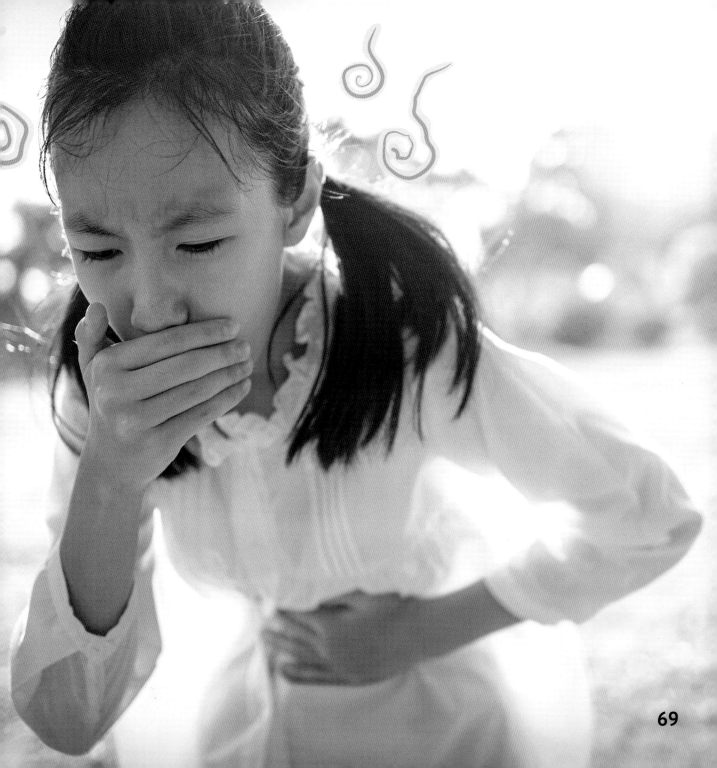

Why can't babies eat normal food?

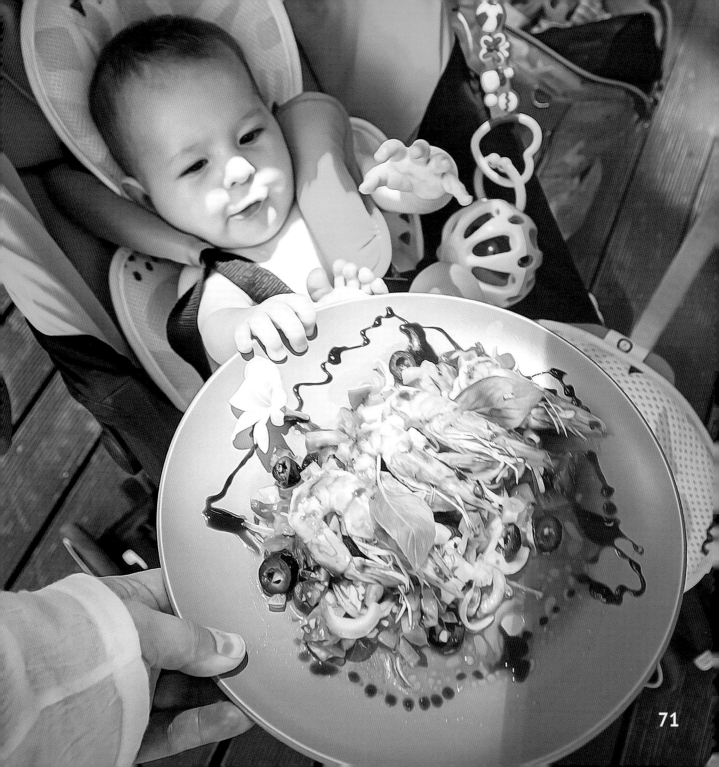

A baby may not be developed enough to swallow solid food.

Babies can't chew food very well, either, thanks to their lack of teeth. Plus, who wants to airplane a chicken drumstick?

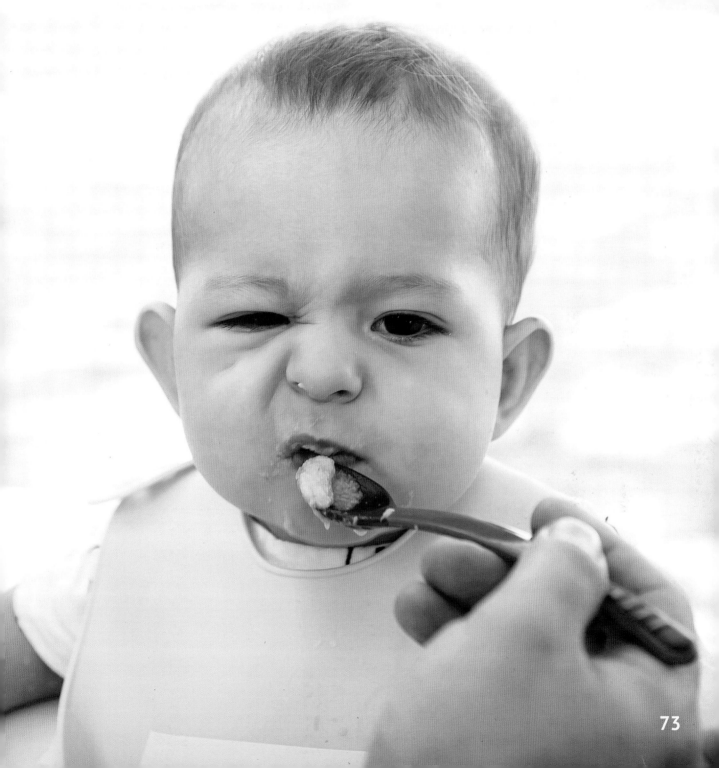

What does grass eat?

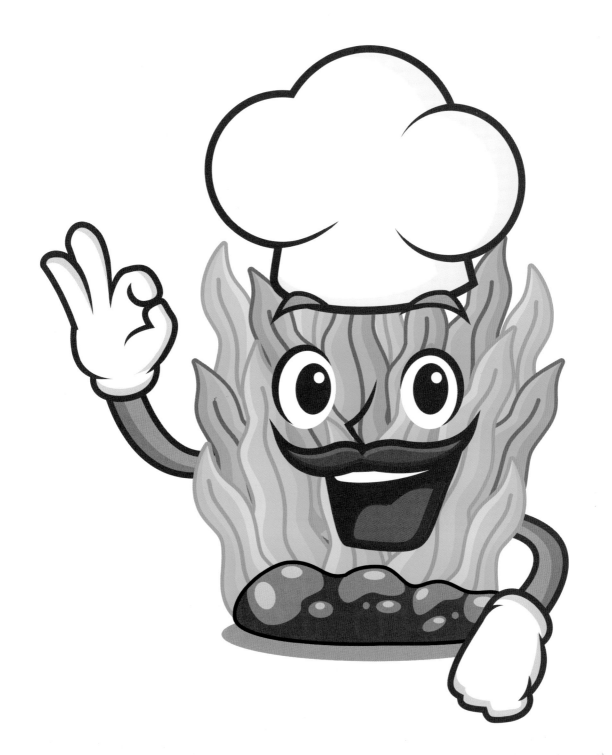

Water and sunshine.

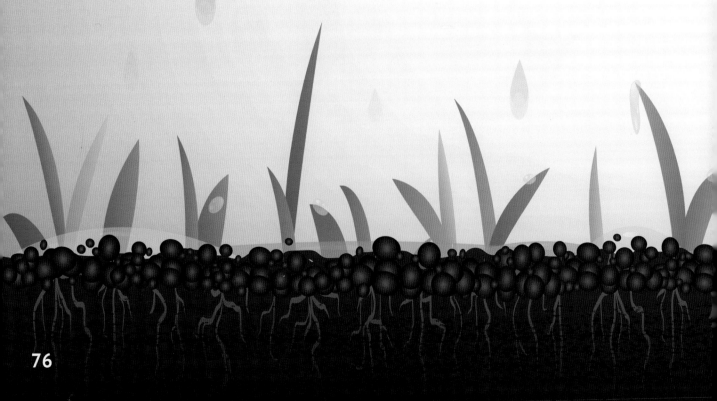

Grass has threadlike roots that absorb water and nutrients from the soil. Grasses also make their own food using sunlight. Humans eat more grass than you might think. Such cereal grasses as wheat, oats, barley, and corn, for example, are used to make bread.

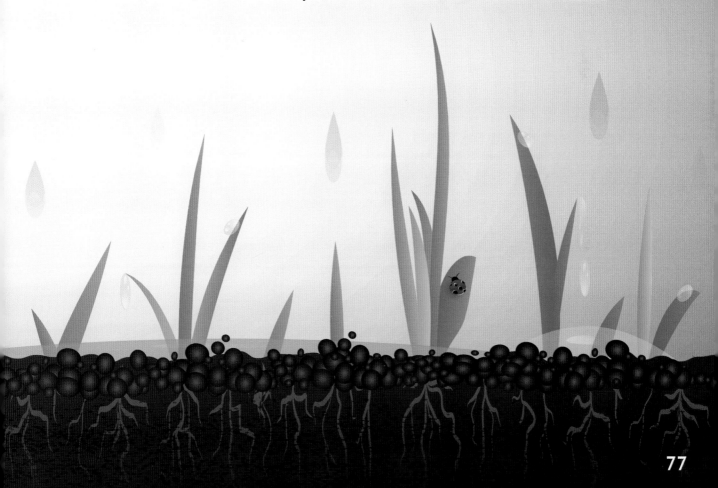

How do tomatoes

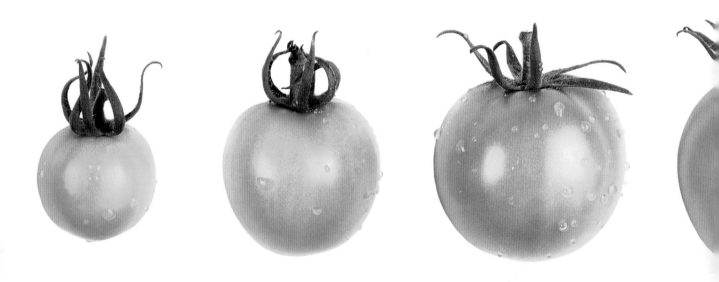

turn red?

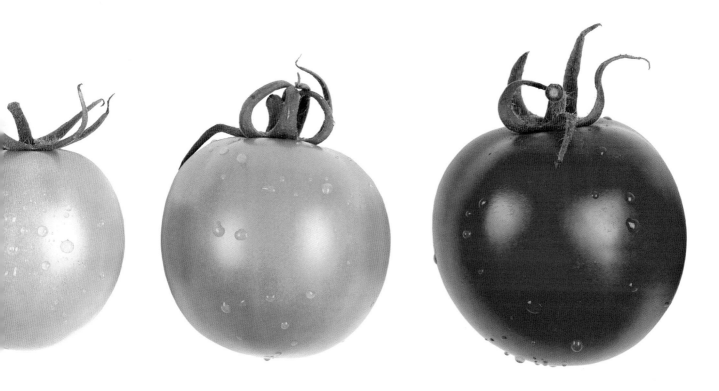

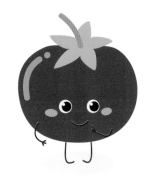

They get embarrassed when people mistake them for a vegetable.

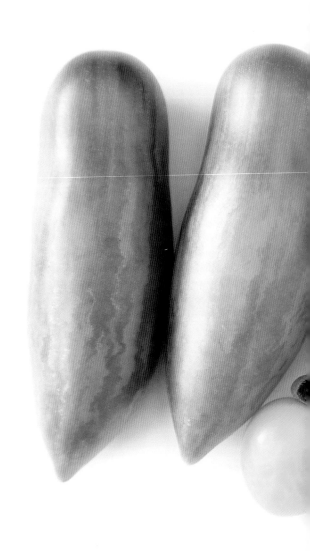

Tomatoes are green at first, but most turn red as they ripen. Some varieties don't turn red at all. Some are green, yellow, or even purple.

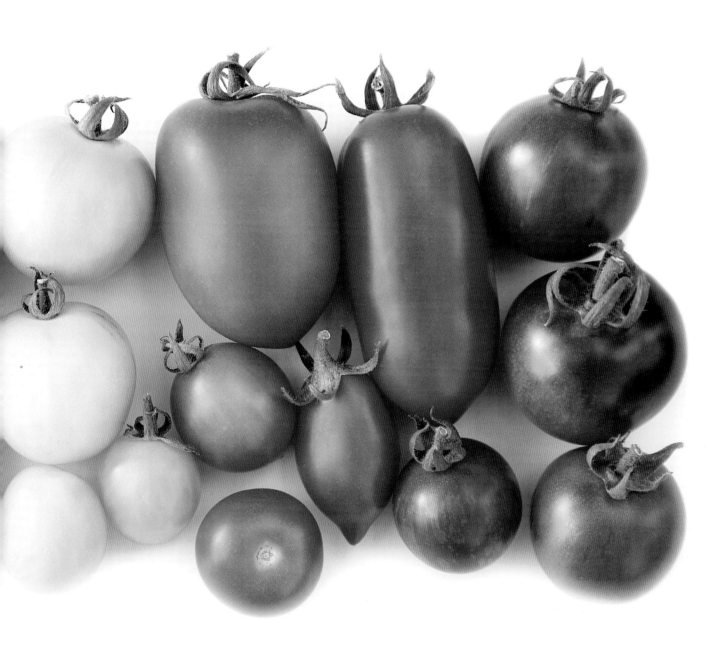

Why are some people allergic to certain foods?

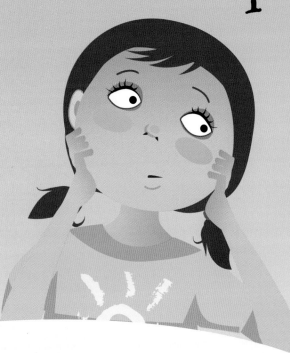
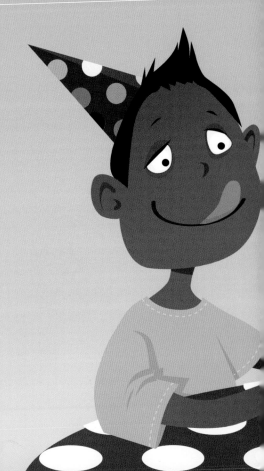

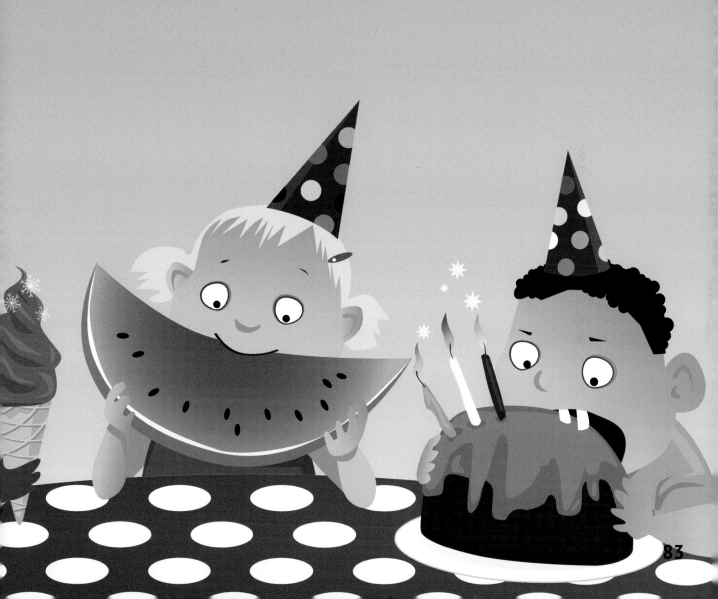

83

Because their immune systems
can't stand
some substances.

The immune system protects the body by attacking harmful things such as bacteria and viruses. You become allergic to something when the immune system mistakes it for something dangerous. Things that may cause allergies include peanuts, shellfish, and little brothers (just kidding).

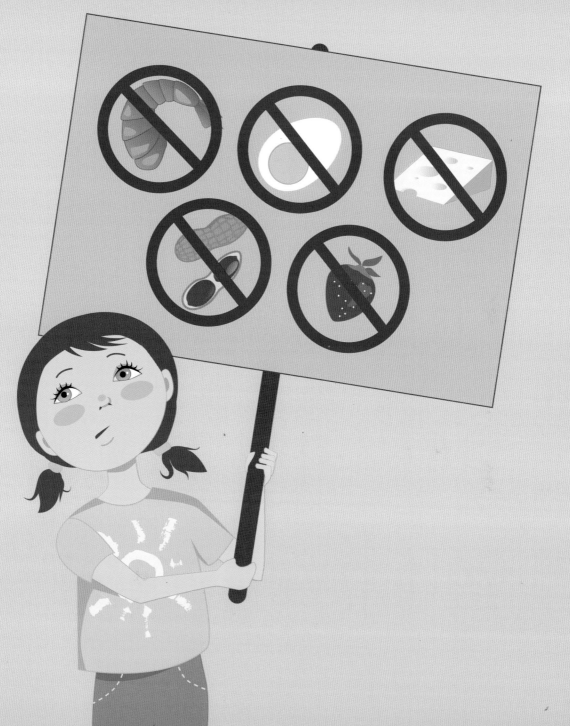

Can being a vegetarian actually make you live longer?

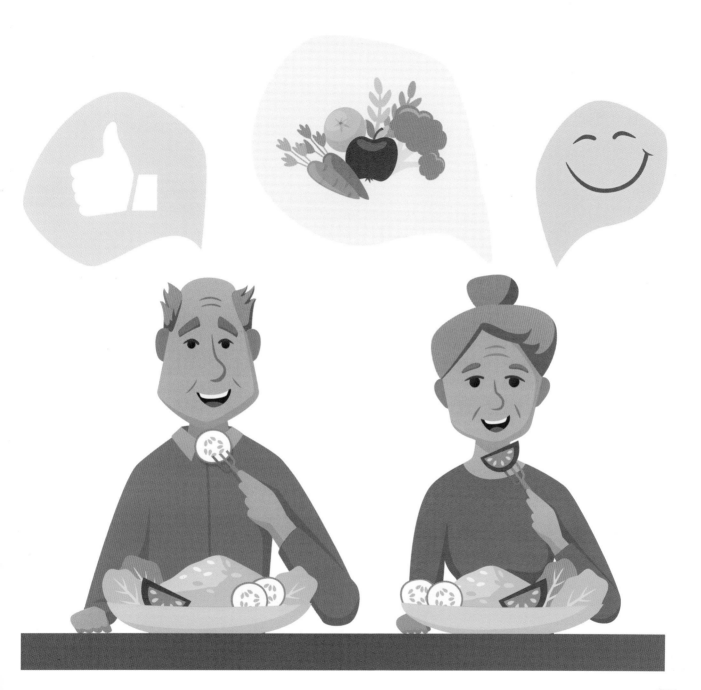

Some people think so.

When it comes to antioxidants, vegetarians have got meat-eaters **beet.** Antioxidants are chemicals that protect cells from damage. Vegetarians also benefit from healthy compounds called *phytochemicals.* They might help vegetarians live longer.

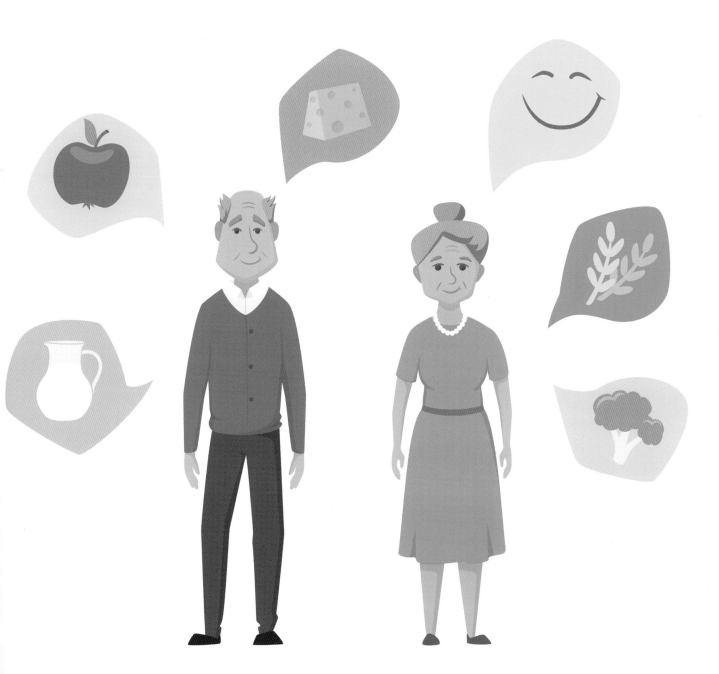

Where is the peanut gallery?

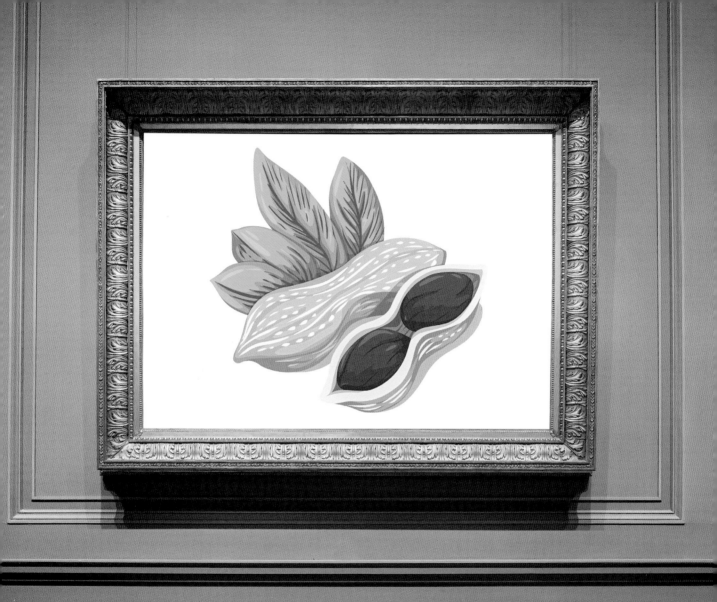

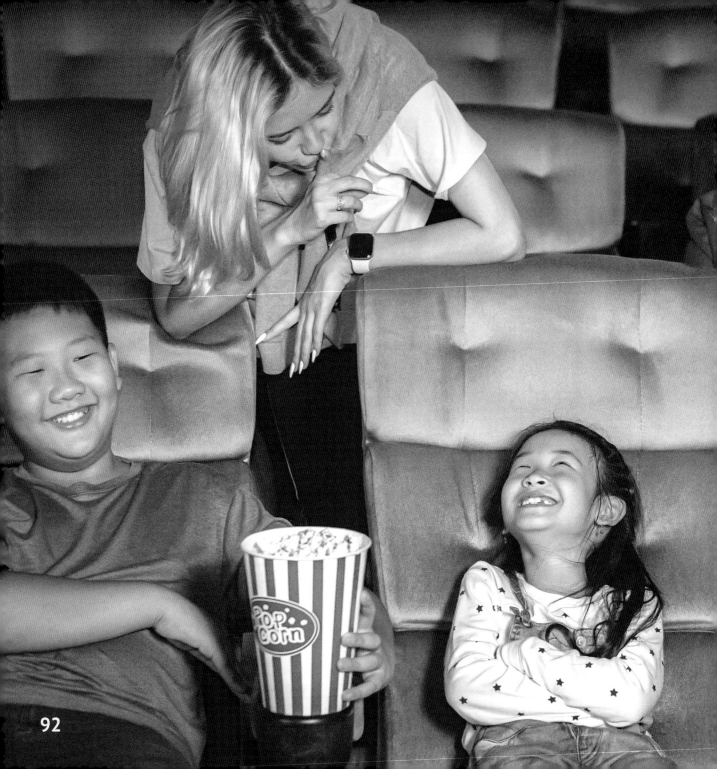

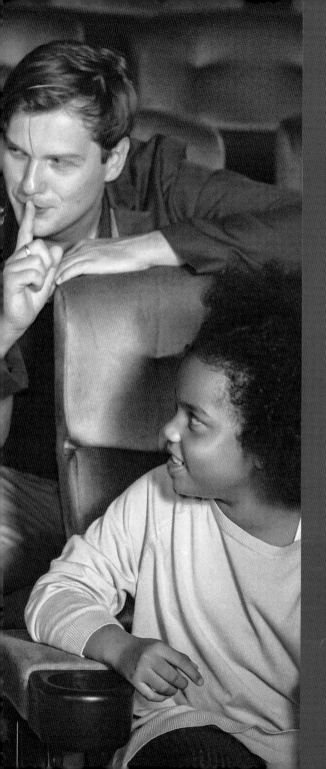

When people say, "No comments from the peanut gallery," they are not referring to a famous museum celebrating the humble-yet-powerful peanut. The phrase refers to the cheap seats of a theatre. There, audience members would loudly yell and throw peanuts at acts they didn't like. But, peanuts are for eating, not throwing!

93

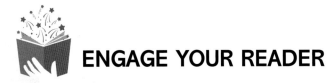

ENGAGE YOUR READER

GUIDED READING PROMPTS

Before Reading

- Allow readers to scan the text and discuss what they notice so far. Highlight the Question-and-Answer structure of this text and discuss a plan for reading.
- Explain the literacy skill: *Asking and answering questions helps us learn new information about the world around us! We can think more critically and deeply when we use higher levels of questions.*

During Reading

- Read each question and provide time to discuss readers' answers before turning the page to learn the facts. Did any of the facts surprise your readers?
- Practice the skills of retelling and summarizing by prompting your readers to rephrase the answer found in the text in their own words.
- Encourage readers to ask their own questions: *Now that you know this, what other related questions do you have?*

After Reading

- Prompt your readers to connect, extend, and challenge their thinking about the text:
  - *How are these ideas connected to what you already knew?*
  - *What new ideas did you get that extended or pushed your thinking in new directions?*
  - *What ideas are still challenging you? What questions, wonders, or puzzles do you still have?*

LOOK BACK!

What other examples of Level 1, 2, and 3 questions can you find in this text?

COMMON CORE CONNECTIONS

These questions and tasks align with the following Common Core College and Career Readiness Anchor Standards for Reading:

- CCSS.ELA-Literacy.CCRA.R.1
- CCSS.ELA-Literacy.CCRA.R.4
- CCSS.ELA-Literacy.CCRA.R.5
- CCSS.ELA-Literacy.CCRA.R.10

LITERACY SKILL

Asking and answering high level questions helps us think critically!

Check out Costa's Levels of Questioning:

- Level 1 – basic questions that help you <u>gather</u> information
    - Includes defining, describing, and identifying
- Level 2 – intermediate questions that help you <u>process</u> information
    - Includes explaining, inferring, and classifying
- Level 3 – more advanced questions that help you <u>apply</u> information
    - Includes evaluating, generalizing, and speculating

Examples from the text:

- Level 1 – p. 6-9 – Who invented candy?
- Level 2 – p. 78-81 – How do tomatoes turn red?
- Level 3 – p. 54-57 – How good is lava at popping popcorn?

EXTEND THROUGH WRITING

Ask your readers what they wonder about food and eating.

- Have readers determine whether their questions involve gathering, processing, or applying information.
- Direct readers to create at least two Level 1, 2, and 3 questions about food and eating.
- Challenge readers to research, determine the answers, and record them alongside the questions.

MORE WAYS TO ENGAGE!

- Create a question web by drawing a spider web on a piece of paper or by creating one out of yarn or rope. Encourage readers to practice asking questions while reading. When they come to a question, they can write it on a sticky note and add it to the web! Revisit these questions, determine their Costa's Level of Questioning, and work to find the answers together.
- Discuss what information in the book really took your readers by surprise and why they were not expecting that answer.

World Book, Inc.
180 North LaSalle Street
Suite 900
Chicago, Illinois 60601
USA

For information about other "Answer Me This, World Book" titles, as well as other World Book print and digital publications, please go to www.worldbook.com.

For information about other World Book publications, call 1-800-WORLDBK (967-5325).

For information about sales to schools and libraries, call 1-800-975-3250 (United States) or 1-800-837-5365 (Canada).

Library of Congress Cataloging-in-Publication Data for this volume has been applied for.

Answer Me This, World Book
ISBN: 978-0-7166-4675-4 (set, hc.)

Can I eat a banana peel?
World Book answers your questions about food and eating
ISBN: 978-0-7166-4678-5 (hc.)

Also available as:
ISBN: 978-0-7166-4688-4 (e-book)

Printed in India by Thomson Press (India) Limited,
Uttar Pradesh, India
1st printing June 2022

Staff

Editorial

Writer
Madeline King

Senior Manager, New Content
Jeff De La Rosa

Manager, New Product
Nick Kilzer

Senior Content Creator
William D. Adams

Curriculum Designer
Caroline Davidson

Proofreader
Nathaniel Lindstrom

Graphics and Design

Senior Visual
Communications Designer
Melanie Bender

Coordinator, Design Development
and Production
Brenda Tropinski

Senior Media Editor
Rosalia Bledsoe

Acknowledgments

Cover: © PV productions/Shutterstock; © Jocularity Art/Shutterstock;
    © dedMazay/Shutterstock
2-24 © Shutterstock
25   © Edward Parker, Alamy Images
26-33 © Shutterstock
34-36 NASA/Goddard/Lunar Reconnaissance Orbiter; © Studiostoks/Shutterstock
37-46 © Shutterstock
49   © Maurizio De Angelis, Science Photo Library
50-94 © Shutterstock